Surviving Cancer

One Patient's Story Of Resilience And Hope

Dr. Jane Frey

Table Of Contents

Conclusion

- Progress In Cancer Treatment:
- The Importance of Multidisciplinary Care:
- The Importance Of Support
- Financial Support
- The Importance Of Advocacy
- Resilience And Hope

Introduction

Cancer is a devastating disease that affects millions of people around the world every year. It is a condition that not only affects the physical health of a person but also their mental and emotional well-being.

Being diagnosed with cancer is a life-changing event that can leave individuals feeling helpless, scared, and overwhelmed. However, many individuals have shown that it is possible to survive cancer and come out stronger on the other side.

Surviving Cancer: One Patient's Story of Resilience and Hope" is a book that chronicles the journey of one such individual who battled cancer and emerged victorious.

This book tells the story of a cancer survivor who found the strength and resilience to overcome the challenges of this debilitating disease.

The author of this book is a cancer survivor who has undergone the grueling process of cancer treatment and emerged on the other side. Through their own experience, the author shares their journey of battling cancer, the emotional and physical challenges that they faced, and how they managed to overcome these obstacles.

The book is divided into several chapters that cover different aspects of the author's journey. The first chapter introduces the author and their background before they were diagnosed with cancer. The subsequent chapters cover the diagnosis, treatment, and recovery process, as well as the emotional and mental toll that cancer can take on a person.

The final chapter focuses on the author's life after cancer, and how they have managed to move forward and find hope and meaning in their life.

The author's journey is not only inspiring, but it also provides a unique perspective on what it means to live with and survive cancer.

They share their personal experiences and insights on how to deal with the physical and emotional challenges that come with a cancer diagnosis. The author also provides practical advice on how to cope with the effects of cancer treatment, such as fatigue, nausea, and pain.

One of the key themes of the book is resilience. The author emphasizes the importance of being resilient and having a positive attitude when facing cancer.

They explain how they were able to find the strength to persevere through the difficult times and how having a positive mindset helped them cope with the challenges of cancer treatment.

Another important theme of the book is hope. The author believes that hope is essential for anyone battling cancer, and they share how they were able to find hope amid their diagnosis and treatment. They provide insights on how to stay hopeful and positive even in the darkest of times.

Overall, "Surviving Cancer: One Patient's Story of Resilience and Hope" is a powerful and inspiring book that offers hope and encouragement to anyone who is currently battling cancer or has a loved one who is.

It is a book that provides a unique perspective on what it means to live with cancer and shows that it is possible to overcome the challenges of this disease.

The author's journey is a testament to the power of resilience and hope, and their story will undoubtedly inspire and motivate others who are facing similar challenges.

Chapter One

Diagnosis And Treatment

Cancer is a group of diseases characterized by the abnormal and uncontrolled growth of cells that have the potential to invade and spread to other parts of the body. It is a complex and multifaceted disease that affects millions of people around the world each year.

The diagnosis of cancer can be a devastating experience for patients, their families, and loved ones. The shock of the diagnosis can be overwhelming, and it can take time to come to terms with the news.

However, early detection and timely treatment can significantly improve the chances of successful treatment and recovery.

The Shock Of The Diagnosis

A cancer diagnosis can be a life-altering event that can evoke a range of emotions, from shock and disbelief to anger, fear, and depression. The news can be overwhelming, and it is normal to feel overwhelmed, scared, and uncertain about what the future holds.

Coping with a cancer diagnosis can be challenging, and it is important to take care of your emotional, mental, and physical health during this time.

It is essential to find support during this time, whether it be from family, friends, or a support group. It can also be helpful to seek professional counseling or therapy to help process the emotions and feelings that come with a cancer diagnosis.

Educating oneself about the disease, treatment options, and potential outcomes can also help alleviate anxiety and empower patients to make informed decisions about their care.

Finding The Right Treatment

The treatment of cancer depends on the type, stage, and location of the cancer, as well as the patient's overall health and medical history.

Treatment options may include surgery, chemotherapy, radiation therapy, targeted therapy, immunotherapy, or a combination of these approaches.

Surgery is often the first-line treatment for many types of cancer. It involves removing the cancerous tissue from the body, and it may be used alone or in combination with other treatments.

Chemotherapy is a systemic treatment that uses drugs to kill cancer cells throughout the body. It may be administered orally or intravenously and can cause side effects such as nausea, vomiting, hair loss, and fatigue.

Radiation therapy uses high-energy radiation to kill cancer cells. It may be used alone or in combination with other treatments and can cause side effects such as skin irritation, fatigue, and nausea.

Targeted therapy is a type of treatment that uses drugs to specifically target cancer cells while leaving healthy cells unharmed. It may be used alone or in combination with other treatments and can cause side effects such as diarrhea, skin rash, and fatigue.

Immunotherapy is a newer approach to cancer treatment that uses drugs to stimulate the body's immune system to recognize and attack cancer cells.

It may be used alone or in combination with other treatments and can cause side effects such as fatigue, fever, and nausea.

It is essential to work closely with a team of healthcare professionals, including an oncologist, surgeon, radiation oncologist, and other specialists, to determine the most appropriate treatment plan for each patient. Treatment decisions should take into account the patient's individual needs and preferences, as well as potential risks and benefits.

Coping With The Side Effects

Many cancer treatments can cause side effects that can affect a patient's quality of life. Coping with these side effects can be challenging, but some strategies can help.

For example, eating a healthy diet and staying hydrated can help manage side effects such as nausea and fatigue. Gentle exercises, such as walking or yoga, can help improve energy levels and mood. Supportive care, such as pain management and palliative care, can also help alleviate symptoms and improve quality of life.

It is important to communicate with your healthcare team about any side effects or concerns you may have. They can offer guidance and support to help manage side effects and improve overall well-being

A cancer diagnosis can be overwhelming, but with early detection and appropriate treatment, many people can survive and even thrive after cancer.

Coping with the shock of a cancer diagnosis, finding the right treatment, and managing the side effects can be challenging, but it is essential to seek support from healthcare professionals, family, friends, and support groups.

Chapter Two

Support System

Cancer is a life-altering disease that affects millions of people worldwide. The physical, emotional, and psychological impact of cancer can be overwhelming for both the patient and their loved ones.However, with the support of family, friends, and healthcare professionals, people with cancer can cope better and improve their quality of life. In this essay, we will explore the various support systems available for people with cancer, including the importance of family and friends, connecting with other survivors, and seeking professional help.

Importance Of Family And Friends

Family and friends are an essential source of support for people with cancer. They provide emotional support, practical assistance, and a sense of comfort during the cancer journey.

Family members can help with daily activities such as cooking, cleaning, and running errands, giving the patient more time to focus on their treatment and recovery.

Moreover, family and friends offer emotional support, which is vital for people with cancer. They provide a listening ear, offer words of encouragement, and help the patient to maintain a positive outlook.

Research has shown that people with strong social support tend to have better mental and physical health outcomes than those without.

Furthermore, family and friends can help people with cancer to make important treatment decisions. They can attend medical appointments with the patient, ask questions, and offer insights into the patient's preferences and needs. This support can help patients feel more confident in their treatment decisions, leading to better outcomes.

Connecting With Other Survivors

Connecting with other cancer survivors can be a valuable source of support for people with cancer.

Survivors can offer unique insights into the cancer journey, providing a sense of community and understanding that is difficult to find elsewhere. They can share their experiences, offer tips and advice, and provide hope and encouragement to others going through a similar experience.

There are many ways to connect with other cancer survivors, including support groups, online forums, and social media groups.

Support groups are often facilitated by healthcare professionals and provide a safe and supportive space for patients and their loved ones to share their experiences. Online forums and social media groups offer a convenient way to connect with others from the comfort of home.

Connecting with other survivors can also help people with cancer to feel less alone and isolated. Cancer can be a lonely journey, but connecting with others who understand the experience can provide a sense of belonging and reduce feelings of isolation.

Seeking Professional Help

Professional help is another important support system for people with cancer. Healthcare professionals such as doctors, nurses, and social workers can provide expert medical care, emotional support, and practical assistance.

They can help patients navigate the complex healthcare system, provide information about treatment options, and offer advice on managing symptoms and side effects.

Healthcare professionals can also provide emotional support to patients and their loved ones. They can help patients cope with the emotional impact of cancer, including anxiety, depression, and fear.

They can provide counseling, refer patients to mental health professionals, and offer support groups and other resources.

Moreover, healthcare professionals can help patients with cancer to manage their physical symptoms and side effects. They can prescribe medications, offer dietary advice, and provide exercise programs to help patients manage their symptoms and improve their overall well-being.

Cancer is a challenging disease that requires a comprehensive support system to help patients cope and improve their quality of life. Family and friends are an essential source of emotional and practical support while connecting with other survivors can provide a sense of community and belonging. Seeking professional help from healthcare professionals can also provide expert medical care, emotional support, and practical assistance.

Together, these support systems can help people with cancer to navigate the complex journey of cancer, cope with the emotional and physical impact of the disease, and improve their overall well-being.

Chapter Three

Mental And Emotional Health

People living with cancer face many challenges, including anxiety, depression, fear of recurrence, and many other mental and emotional health issues.

In this article, we will explore the mental and emotional health of people living with cancer, how to deal with anxiety and depression, ways to stay positive, and how to manage the fear of recurrence.

Mental And Emotional Health Of People Living With Cancer

Being diagnosed with cancer can have a significant impact on an individual's mental and emotional health.

Fear, anxiety, sadness, and anger are all common emotions that can arise during this difficult time. The stress of cancer and its treatment can also have physical effects, such as fatigue, insomnia, and changes in appetite.

It is important to understand that these emotions are normal and that there are many ways to manage them.

Talking to a mental health professional, such as a counselor or therapist, can help manage provideotions and provide emotional support. Joining a support group with others who are going through a similar experience can also provide a sense of community and support.

Dealing With Anxiety And Depression

Anxiety and depression are common mental health issues experienced by people living with cancer. Anxiety can manifest as worry, fear, or panic, while depression can result in feelings of sadness, hopelessness, and loss of interest in activities. These mental health issues can be difficult to manage, but many strategies can help.

One effective strategy for managing anxiety and depression is cognitive-behavioral therapy (CBT). This type of therapy focuses on identifying negative thought patterns and developing skills to change them. CBT can be done with a therapist or on one's own with the help of self-help resources.

Another effective strategy for managing anxiety and depression is mindfulness meditation. This practice involves paying attention to the present moment without judgment. Mindfulness can help individuals become more aware of their thoughts and feelings and can reduce anxiety and depression symptoms.

Exercise is also an effective way to manage anxiety and depression. Regular exercise has been shown to reduce symptoms of anxiety and depression, and can also improve physical health. Exercise can be done in many forms, such as walking, swimming, or yoga.

Finding Ways To o Stay Positive

Staying positive can be a challenge for people living with cancer, but it is an important aspect of mental and emotional health. Maintaining a positive outlook can improve quality of life and help individuals cope with the challenges of cancer treatment. There are many ways to stay positive, including:

Finding joy in everyday activities: Engaging in activities that bring joy, such as spending time with loved ones, listening to music, or reading a good book, can help improve mood and promote positivity.

Practicing gratitude: Focusing on the positive aspects of life and expressing gratitude for them can help shift focus away from negative thoughts and emotions.

Setting realistic goals: Setting achievable goals, such as completing a project or learning a new skill, can provide a sense of accomplishment and boost self-esteem.

Engaging in creative activities: Creative activities, such as painting or writing, can help individuals express their emotions and promote positivity.

Managing Fear Of Recurrence

The fear of recurrence is a common concern for people living with cancer. This fear can be overwhelming and can have a significant impact on mental and emotional health. Many strategies can help manage this fear, including:

Staying informed: Learning about the risk of recurrence and the steps that can be taken to reduce this risk can help individuals feel more in control and reduce anxiety.

Practicing self-care: Engaging in activities that promote physical and emotional health, such as exercise, mindfulness, and socializing, can help reduce anxiety and promote overall well-being, which can help manage the fear of recurrence.

Seeking support: Talking to a mental health professional, joining a support group, or reaching out to friends and family for support can help individuals cope with the fear of recurrence and provide emotional support.

Developing coping strategies: Developing coping strategies, such as positive self-talk, relaxation techniques, and problem-solving skills, can help individuals manage the fear of recurrence and reduce anxiety.

Developing a plan: Developing a plan with healthcare providers to monitor for recurrence and take proactive steps if necessary can help individuals feel more in control and reduce anxiety.

The mental and emotional health of people living with cancer is a critical aspect of overall well-being. The challenges of cancer can impact an individual's mental and emotional health, but many strategies can help manage anxiety, depression, and the fear of recurrence.

It is important to seek support and develop coping strategies to promote positive mental and emotional health.

With proper care and support, individuals living with cancer can improve their mental and emotional well-being and lead fulfilling lives.

Chapter Four

Lifestyle Changes

In addition to the physical symptoms, cancer can also have a significant impact on a person's mental and emotional well-being. As such, people living with cancer often need to make significant lifestyle changes to help manage their condition.

In this article, we will explore some of the lifestyle changes that people with cancer can make to improve their overall health and well-being. We will specifically discuss exercise and physical activity, nutrition and diet, and alternative therapies.

Exercise And Physical Activity

One of the most important lifestyle changes that people with cancer can make is to incorporate regular exercise and physical activity into their routine.

Exercise has been shown to have numerous health benefits, including reducing the risk of cardiovascular disease, improving bone density, and boosting the immune system. For people with cancer, exercise can also help to alleviate many of the symptoms associated with the disease and its treatment.

There are many different types of exercise that people with cancer can engage in, depending on their individual needs and preferences.

For example, some people may prefer low-impact activities such as yoga or tai chi, while others may enjoy more vigorous activities like running or weight lifting. Whatever the activity, it is important to start slowly and gradually increase the intensity and duration of exercise over time.

In addition to the physical benefits, exercise can also have a positive impact on a person's mental and emotional well-being. Many people with cancer report feeling more energized and less fatigued after engaging in regular exercise, which can help to improve their overall quality of life.

Exercise has also been shown to have a positive effect on mood and anxiety, helping people to feel more relaxed and less stressed.

Nutrition And Diet

Another important lifestyle change that people with cancer can make is to improve their nutrition and diet. Eating a healthy and balanced diet can help to boost the immune system, improve energy levels, and promote overall health and well-being.

For people with cancer, good nutrition is especially important as it can help to manage some of the side effects of cancer treatment, such as nausea, vomiting, and fatigue.

A healthy diet for people with cancer should include plenty of fruits and vegetables, whole grains, lean proteins, and healthy fats. It is also important to stay hydrated by drinking plenty of water and other fluids throughout the day.

Some people with cancer may also benefit from working with a registered dietitian to develop a personalized nutrition plan based on their individual needs and preferences.

In addition to eating a healthy diet, people with cancer may also benefit from taking supplements or other dietary interventions. For example, some studies have shown that taking omega-3 fatty acid supplements may help to reduce inflammation and improve overall health in people with cancer.

Other supplements, such as vitamin D and probiotics, may also have potential benefits for people with cancer, although more research is needed in these areas.

Alternative Therapies:

In addition to exercise and nutrition, there are also many alternative therapies that people with cancer may find helpful.

Alternative therapies are often used in conjunction with traditional cancer treatments and can help to manage some of the physical and emotional symptoms associated with cancer.

Some examples of alternative therapies that people with cancer may find helpful include acupuncture, massage therapy, and meditation. Acupuncture has been shown to help alleviate pain, nausea, and other symptoms associated with cancer treatment.

Massage therapy can help to reduce stress and promote relaxation, while meditation can help to improve mental and emotional well-being.

Other alternative therapies that may be helpful for people with cancer include herbal remedies, aromatherapy, and hypnotherapy. However, it is important to note that not all alternative therapies are backed by scientific evidence, and some may even be harmful if not used properly.

As such, it is important to speak with a healthcare provider before trying any alternative therapies, and to ensure that they are safe and appropriate for your individual needs and medical history.

Living with cancer can be challenging, but there are many lifestyle changes that people with cancer can make to improve their overall health and well-being.

Exercise and physical activity can help to manage symptoms and improve mental and emotional well-being, while a healthy diet can boost the immune system and help manage the side effects of treatment.

Alternative therapies can also help manage and improve the overall quality of life, but it is important to ensure that they are safe and appropriate for your individual needs and medical history.

By making these lifestyle changes, people with cancer can take control of their health and improve their chances of a successful recovery.

Chapter Five

Finding Meaning And Purpose

A cancer diagnosis can be a life-changing event for both the patient and their loved ones. It can be a challenging experience, filled with uncertainty, fear, and anxiety. It is a time when one's life is often put on hold, and the focus is solely on getting through treatment and recovery.

However, amidst the chaos, finding meaning and purpose can be a powerful way to help individuals living with cancer navigate this journey with resilience and hope.

This essay explores how people living with cancer can re-evaluate their priorities, rediscover passions and hobbies, and give back to the cancer community to find meaning and purpose in their lives.

Re-evaluating Priorities

A cancer diagnosis often prompts individuals to re-evaluate their priorities and consider what is most important in their lives. It can help them gain perspective on what matters and focus their energy on things that bring them joy and fulfillment.

For some, this may mean spending more time with family and friends, while for others, it may mean focusing on personal growth and development.

Either way, the process of re-evaluating priorities can help individuals find a sense of purpose and direction in their lives.

Rediscovering Passions And Hobbies

Cancer treatments can be challenging and often leave individuals feeling tired and unmotivated. However, rediscovering passions and hobbies can be an excellent way to find joy and meaning in life.

Pursuing activities that bring pleasure and fulfillment can provide a much-needed break from the stress of treatment and create a sense of normalcy in one's life.

For example, taking up a new hobby like painting, writing, or photography can be a therapeutic way to express emotions and cope with the challenges of cancer.

Giving Back To The Cancer Community

Many people living with cancer find purpose and meaning by giving back to the cancer community.

This may involve volunteering with local organizations, participating in fundraising events, or sharing their experiences with others who are going through a similar journey.

Not only does this help individuals find a sense of purpose and meaning, but it can also provide a sense of empowerment and control in a situation that often feels overwhelming and uncontrollable.

Conclusion

Cancer is a leading cause of death worldwide, with over 9.6 million deaths in 2018 alone. The incidence of cancer is on the rise globally, with an estimated 18.1 million new cases in 2018. Cancer affects individuals and their families both physically and emotionally, with significant economic and social consequences.

The journey of cancer is often long and challenging, with patients and their loved ones experiencing physical, emotional, and financial stress. However, with modern treatments and a multidisciplinary approach to care, more individuals are surviving cancer and leading fulfilling lives.

As we move forward in the fight against cancer, it is essential to reflect on the progress made, the challenges that still exist, and the opportunities to improve the lives of people living with cancer. In this essay, we will discuss the resilience and hope needed to move forward in the fight against cancer.

Progress In Cancer Treatment:

The past few decades have seen significant progress in the diagnosis and treatment of cancer. Advances in technology and research have led to new treatment options, including targeted therapies, immunotherapies, and precision medicine.

These treatments have improved outcomes and quality of life for many cancer patients. Targeted therapies are designed to attack specific cancer cells' vulnerabilities, leading to fewer side effects than traditional chemotherapy.

Immunotherapies work by harnessing the power of the body's immune system to fight cancer cells. Precision medicine involves using genomic and molecular data to personalize treatment for each patient.

In addition to new treatment options, there have been significant improvements in cancer screening and early detection. Early detection is crucial in improving survival rates for many cancers, including breast, colon, and cervical cancer.

The Importance of Multidisciplinary Care:

Cancer treatment is not a one-size-fits-all approach. The complex nature of cancer requires a multidisciplinary approach to care. Multidisciplinary care involves a team of healthcare professionals working together to provide the best possible care for the patient.

The team may include medical oncologists, radiation oncologists, surgeons, nurses, social workers, and other healthcare professionals. This team approach ensures that patients receive comprehensive care that addresses their physical, emotional, and social needs.

The Importance Of Support

Cancer affects not only the individual but also their family and loved ones. The emotional toll of cancer can be significant, and it is essential to have a strong support system in place. Support can come from many sources, including family, friends, support groups, and mental health professionals.

Support groups provide a safe and supportive environment for individuals to share their experiences with others who have gone through similar experiences. These groups can help reduce feelings of isolation and provide emotional support.

Mental health professionals, such as psychologists and psychiatrists, can also provide support for individuals experiencing emotional distress related to cancer. They can provide counseling and therapy to help individuals cope with the stress and anxiety associated with cancer.

Financial Support

Cancer treatment can be expensive, and the cost of care can be a significant source of stress for individuals and their families. Many cancer patients face financial difficulties, such as lost income, medical bills, and transportation costs.

There are many organizations and resources available to provide financial support for cancer patients. These resources include patient assistance programs, cancer-specific organizations, and government programs.

Patient assistance programs offer financial assistance to patients who cannot afford their medications or other healthcare costs.

Cancer-specific organizations provide financial assistance, counseling, and other resources to cancer patients and their families. Government programs, such as Medicare and Medicaid, also provide financial assistance to eligible individuals.

The Importance Of Advocacy

Advocacy plays a critical role in the fight against cancer. Advocacy involves raising awareness, promoting research, and influencing policy. Cancer advocacy groups work to raise awareness about the importance of cancer prevention and early detection. They also promote research to develop new treatments and improve the quality of life for cancer patients.

Advocacy groups also play a crucial role in influencing policy related to cancer care and research. They advocate for increased funding for cancer research, improved access to care, and policies that support cancer patients and their families.

By advocating for change, cancer advocacy groups help ensure that the needs of cancer patients are heard and addressed. They empower individuals and communities to make a difference in the fight against cancer.

Resilience And Hope

Cancer is a challenging disease, but individuals and their families have shown incredible resilience in the face of adversity.

Resilience involves the ability to adapt and cope with difficult situations, and cancer patients and their families demonstrate this resilience every day.

Resilience is not something that comes naturally, but it can be developed through the support of others, the ability to find meaning in difficult situations, and the belief in one's ability to overcome challenges.

Hope is also an essential aspect of the cancer journey. Hope involves the belief that things will get better and that there is a future worth fighting for.

Hope can come from many sources, including the support of loved ones, the belief in one's ability to overcome challenges, and the promise of new treatments and advances in cancer care.

The fight against cancer requires resilience, hope, and a multidisciplinary approach to care. Significant progress has been made in the diagnosis and treatment of cancer, and individuals are surviving cancer and leading fulfilling lives.

However, challenges still exist, including the high cost of care, the emotional toll of cancer, and the need for continued research and advocacy. It is essential to continue to work together to address these challenges and improve the lives of individuals living with cancer.

Through support, advocacy, and a belief in the power of hope and resilience, we can move forward in the fight against cancer with the knowledge that progress is possible and that a brighter future is within reach.

www.ingramcontent.com/pod-product-compliance
Lightning Source LLC
Chambersburg PA
CBHW070851220526
45466CB00005B/1956